I0439857

7 DAY BOMB

LOSE 7 POUNDS IN 7 DAYS

Scott & Naomi Barlow

DAMAGE CONTROL

CONTENTS

ACKNOWLEDGEMENTS

1 THE 7 DAY BOMB   1

2 INTRODUCTION   3

3 THE RIGHT WAY   13

4 RIGHT HERE, RIGHT NOW   16

5 DEFINE YOUR REASON   24

6 7 DAY BOMB MENU   28

7 THE LAW   34

8 7 DAY BOMB STACK   37

9 TIPS, TRICKS & ADVICE   42

10 THE SHIVER SYSTEM   48

11 MOTHER NATURE'S GYM   51

12 WEIGHT LOSS WISDOM   55

13 REALIZE THIS…   75

14 CHANGE YOUR WORLD   79

15 MEDICAL DISCLAIMER   80

ABOUT THE AUTHOR

The 7 Day Bomb was created by husband and wife team Scott & Naomi Barlow from England. They wanted a weight loss hack that could quickly allow you to drop a huge amount of weight before an event such as a holiday or a wedding. Fed up with traditional diets that only took 2-3 pounds off per week they turned themselves into human guinea pigs and the result was the 7 Day Bomb; where you can lose up to 7 pounds in just 7 days. So whether it's a wedding, a holiday, a party or a date – look sharp and drop that weight in just 7 days.

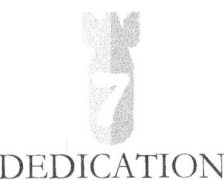

DEDICATION

*"The devil has put a penalty on all things we enjoy in life.
Either we suffer in health or we suffer in soul or we get fat"*
Albert Einstein

I dedicate this book to anyone who has tirelessly fought
the never ending battle against fat. Using the arsenal of
weapons found within this book, may you fight back and
rescue that thin person that the enemy has been holding
hostage for far too along.

ACKNOWLEDGEMENTS

A big thanks goes to my wife Naomi (a diet veteran) for coming along with me on this journey. I would also like to thank Justus von Liebig who invented the mirror – looking at my fat naked body in the mirror has been one of the best motivators!

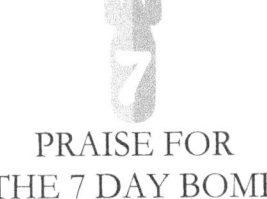

PRAISE FOR
THE 7 DAY BOMB

"When I first answered an online advert to take part in a *new diet* trial I never really believed the claims of losing up to 7 pounds in just 7 days. I have been overweight now for almost 10 years ever since having my kids and have tried almost every diet out there. Although the 7 Day Bomb is tough, it's only 7 days you have to hold out for and this is achievable. In my first week I lost just under 9 pounds and I blew my diet coach away that week at weigh-in."
-   **Sarah White, England**

"I can only praise the 7 Day Bomb for helping me and my bridesmaids lose a combined 6 stone before my wedding this year! We did it together and you can see the results each day by simply standing on the scales. The other little cheats and hacks that Scott has put into the book helps you overcome the struggles of any diet and keeps you motivated. I did the diet before the book was written but have bought the book now and love some of the extra stuff that Scott has added in."
-   **Amy Fisher, England**

"If you don't lose weight on this plan – <u>you will never lose it</u>. I've done this 3 times now and along with another healthy eating plan I have lost nearly 4 stone."
   -   **Bob Harris, Australia**

"After 30 years of living as a single (fat) man after my divorce the 7 Day Bomb helped me kick start a complete life change. I started the 7 Day Bomb when Scott was running the trials and I lost exactly 10 pounds in 7 days. I am now back to a healthy weight and back on the dating scene again!"
   -   **Derek Withe, England**

"I 'drop' the 7 Day 'Bomb' one week before my holiday and then I do it one week after to prevent any damage being done! Definitely a secret for looking great!"
   -   **Gemma Lucas, England**

There are literally hundreds of testimonials and before-and-after photos coming in each day and we will be displaying as many of these as we can on our facebook fan page so ensure you **Like** us and connect with us at **www.facebook.com/7daybomb**

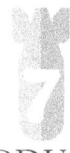

INTRODUCTION

"I have gained and lost the same ten pounds so many times over and over again my cellulite must have déjà vu" **Jane Wagner**

When you're not happy with your body and weight it can be devastating. It robs people of their personality, confidence, style and will even prevent people from doing many things. I wanted to let you know in the first paragraph of this book that I approach the entire topic of losing weight as a serious one. My only concern and objective in writing this book is to help **you lose weight**.

The global weight loss management market was worth $265 billion in 2012. You might say "so what, what's that go to do with me losing weight?" It's important to know that there are a lot of people in this game that are only here to make money. Before I came up with the format of the 7 Day Bomb I must have tried every diet on the market, spent thousands of pounds over the years on "magical" and "secret" diets that just never worked. The only way these diets worked is by putting money each week into the company's pockets that peddled their soups, shakes, bars, videos and exercise equipment etc. You will be pleased to know that this book is not written by yet another doctor or hypnotist but instead a diet veteran who has fought the battle you have been fighting. I am not some superhuman fitness trainer with glowing teeth and a stomach like a washboard. I am the everyday guy who loves food and hates the gym, seriously! I find it easy to gain the pounds and find it extremely hard to lose them. Success at losing weight is a combination of the personal will to lose it and also an effective plan that covers both diet (food) and exercise (doesn't have to be running or a gym membership!) If anything, I am more than qualified to give you advice on losing weight than many of these corporate giants as I have truly been there and rescued my skinny-self back from the jaws of the fat-man inside me!

Losing weight is hard. Whatever weight loss diet or program you have tried and failed at, I can say with absolute confidence that I believe you stand the <u>best chance yet</u> of losing weight joining me on the 7 Day Bomb. Not only have my wife and I lost an incredible amount of weight using the 7 Day Bomb – but we have also worked with nearly 400 hundred people in our testing phase before writing this book. Now these people weren't just anyone off the street. We specifically recruited people who have been trying to lose weight for years, people who believed they had tried everything. We really put the 7 Day Bomb to the test with these people and it was incredible to see people of all ages and backgrounds make breakthrough progress. I am thrilled and excited that you have bought this book and that you are serious about finally shedding that weight – it is my mission to get 1 million people lighter and happier with the 7 Day Bomb.

IN THE BEGINNING

My wife Naomi and I were young, thin and we had just got married. Only two years after getting married and 6 months after the birth of our first child Eva, we realized we had a problem. We were FAT! OK maybe that is a bit extreme but we were not happy with our bodies and so decided to do something about it. Fast forward a year of failed attempts and false starts which usually went something like start on a Monday and fail on a Wednesday we must have tried over 10 different diet plans. Naomi found a group diet plan was working for her where she lost around 1-2 pounds per week and I had opted for a healthy eating plan with exercise and this was also chipping away at about 1-2 pounds per week.

Weight loss was slow! After several months we looked back at our diary (where we wrote down our weekly weight and measurements) and in horror we had only shed around 6 pounds each! How did this happen! Well our busy social lives were too frequent and that meant in the average month we had hen parties, stag do's, weddings, birthday parties, holidays, baby showers, work parties, children's parties, anniversaries and all the other "good food" opportunities such as date night at the cinema! The 1-2 pound loss each week was no match for what we would gain at one of these social events. So we either gained weight or just got back to where we started. It was depressing beyond belief. When Naomi asked her diet coach for advice she was simply told to "cut out the social life"!

So we were at a difficult place. We wanted to lose weight and we were putting in the effort both in terms of the diet/exercise and spending a fortune on all of this diet stuff but as young 'socialites' we didn't want to totally give up our social lives. There had to be a better way. There had to be a way, a plan or system out there that you could follow say one week before an event where you knew you were going to be naughty and it would help you lose the pounds that you were going to put on at the event – a sort of damage control! Counter-balance the huge calorie intake!

Two months later and after reading over 100 blogs, 15 books and watching hours of online videos – there was

<u>nothing out there</u>. So one evening after finding out we had gained yet more pounds than the previous weigh-in we sat down with pen and paper and wrote down what we wanted. Naomi said "I want to lose the weight I would normally put on while on holiday, BUT before I go on holiday".

So what we wanted was a hack, or a cheat that we could do one week before we had a social event. During this hack we could ideally lose as much weight as possible, so when the event came round we could indulge as much as possible but when we got on the scales the following week, we were back to our last weigh-in. No shocking gains to deal with after the event. So simply put – a way where we would lose the weight we would normally gain at such an event. For example, Naomi was losing around 2 pounds per week at her weight loss group, she was at 9 stone 3 pounds and the weekend ahead she was going away on a hen party full of alcohol, chocolates, cake and fast food. The week before, she did the 7 Day Bomb and lost just under 8 pounds. That weekend away Naomi ate and drank until she was full (or close to bursting!) The following week she was at 9 stone 1 pound at her weight loss group. Now that's what we call damage control! All of the damage she had done had been covered during the week before during the 7 Day Bomb.

It was another 8 months before we even got anywhere close to what worked. My research meant me spending long nights and early mornings studying astronauts pre-launch diet plans to weird Christian "water only" fasts. It was shocking to see what some people do to themselves in the name of losing weight quickly. I exchanged emails with American professors, Thai kick boxers, a Tibetan Buddhist monk, the Irish Horse Jockey Association, a World War veteran, an international ballerina and even a plastic surgeon. But one email led the way to me discovering the first version of the 7 Day Bomb and that was from a retired heart surgeon living in California.

DAMAGE CONTROL

Over the period of several weeks I sent over 80 emails to this retired heart surgeon and even got him on a Skype call for an hour to discuss a plan that he used to give his patients who required surgery urgently but were too overweight to go under the knife.

This surgeon would give this diet plan to people who needed an urgent operation or would die! What a motivation for losing weight! But the diet had to ensure this person lost as much weight as possible in a short space of time. So after running over 30 different trials between me and Naomi we took around seven key elements from all the people I spoke with and diet plans ranging from the astronaut and horse jockey diet plans to the heart surgeons diet plan. We also added in some extra elements such as hypothermics where we encourage you to drink ice cold water that drastically lowers your core body temperature meaning your body works extra hard to quickly warm it up – burning an enormous amount of calories in the process (we will fully cover this later in the book).

Our first breakthrough came when we went away on a weeks holiday to Portugal where we spent the week eating everything from Portuguese (as you would expect!) Chinese, Thai, Japanese and the general steaks, to chips and burgers. We lived like kings for the week as we do on every holiday we go on. The difference was that we did the 7 Day Bomb exactly one week before the holiday. When we got back – we jumped straight onto the scales. I had put on 1 pound and Naomi had actually lost 2 pounds from our last "diet weight" reading. Normally after such an event I would have easily put on 6 pounds plus. But we returned happily to our diet regimes as if we had never been away (shush don't tell your weight loss coach!)

After refining the plan yet again (in fact about another 15 times according to Naomi) we decided to share this plan with as many friends and family as possible via our Facebook network. I made a quick Word document with the basics in it and we sent it out. Before we knew it Naomi had requests, questions and praise coming through on her Facebook account. Within weeks we had people we didn't even know emailing asking for advice! It then went viral with people we have never heard of who had got hold of the 7 Day Bomb plan sending us before-and-after photos. After we heard our 100th *"you should write a book and launch this to the world"* we decided we would. The results were just incredible. But then something weird happened.

We initially designed the 7 Day Bomb as a damage control system (and not a diet plan) that you would bolt onto an existing diet plan. You would simply pull it out and implement it one week before a social event such as a wedding or holiday where you know you are going to gain a few pounds from all the indulging. We never expected people to use this as a full time diet plan! This caused issues though as the plan was not sustainable as a full time plan as it is on its own.

You see – the 7 Day Bomb is designed to seriously reduce your calorie intake in such a short space of time that your body kicks into burning some serious fat. But after 7 days (or around the 7th day) your body is burning that much fat that it gets a bit worried and so it then kicks into starvation mode – this is when you stop burning fat as the body prepares to keep as much fat as possible. So we need to be careful if we are using the 7 Day Bomb as a diet; because if you think this weight loss will continue - you will be wrong. So we had to then design a diet plan which incorporates the 7 Day Bomb which is called the **7 Day Bomb Stack**. Don't worry – it's all here in this book, so if you want to use the 7 Day Bomb as a diet plan then we will show you the right way to do it. I must stress though that you must follow our advice if you are using the 7 Day Bomb as a diet plan – get this wrong and you will stop losing weight.

HOW TO USE THIS BOOK

One thing I always remember from reading all of those diet books on my journey to losing weight in the past is how huge the books were! Seriously – I would need to take a couple of weeks to read all of the stuff. Some of these diet books need to lose a few inches in pages! Not sure if this statistic is accurate or not but there is an element of truth that we only take on board between 2-3% of the information from a book, film or talk that we pay attention to. So one of my objectives in writing this book was not to fill it with page filling science that would make no difference to our goal of losing weight. Instead only include what you need to know and structure it in a fun and engaging way.

After several drafts I completely rewrote this book from the heart – I want you to read this as if you were sat across the table from me at a coffee shop (no muffins! Just green teas!) Where I have included a bit of science or research it is only there to try and explain why we do certain things. I found that from the trials those who did not lose significant weight were those who changed elements of the 7 Day Bomb or missed things out or even added stuff! When we drilled down to why they did this it was because they did not agree or understand my reason for doing such as thing. So please – don't skip this information – it's important.

I love seeing people's lives transformed by a simple system that has worked for us. Using social media such as our Facebook fan page (www.facebook.com/7daybomb) there is a community where we all come together every week and join thousands of others on the same journey. I plan to offer competitions, profile before-and-after pictures and also hold Q&A sessions – anything and everything that you need to be successful. I want to see you succeed – I want you to see that you can lose that weight and the 7 Day Bomb is a great way to kick-start a long term life change effort.

One area that Naomi and I struggled with was the 'mind' side of dieting and losing weight. So how our failed efforts over the past several years hampered our initial efforts in the early days when we were trialing the 7 Day Bomb. So I am also going to invest some time before we hit the nuts and bolts of the 7 Day Bomb explaining why you failed in the past and how we can ensure we clear up any lingering thoughts of self-hate or failure attached to dieting and your relationship with food. Please don't see this as spiritual or wishy washy happy clappy stuff or even religious stuff – it is definitely not, it's practical solutions to some of the stuff that prevents us from making real progress. In fact any hat you have on at the moment take it off! Hats are another way of saying pre-judgments. Approach the 7 Day Bomb and this book as an entirely new way of looking at losing weight and changing your life. Be open-minded to this.

So this book is designed that you can read this easily and quickly and then implement it. I cover a bit of background, I challenge the status quo of how we currently see things and do things and then I ask you to step out – make a commitment to taking action.

Here are some reasons why the 7 Day Bomb rocks!

- **It's only 7 days!**

  I remember joining some diet plans and it talks about mapping out a 3-6 month plan. How depressing! I never really got past 2 weeks on these plans. 7 days is relatively easy to stick to. This is the number one reason people mention why they succeeded in this plan.

- **No expensive stuff to buy!**

No sign up fees, no weekly fees, no shakes or meal replacements, no weird exercise equipment to buy.

- **Get started today if you want!**

  Not only do we tell you what to eat, we even provide you with a shopping list for the week and there isn't anything that a normal grocery store wouldn't have. So if you decide today's the day – get to the shops!

- **No sugar crashes!**

  I have the sweetest tooth in the world and I love sugar. Past diets left me in a constant state of feeling I was about to pass out. This diet gives you a daily sugar boost albeit natural sugar via fruit so you still feel good.

- **Immediate results!**

  Step on the scale every day and see the results! Day 2 and you will be motivated to go to day 3 and then day 4 and so on. This is not just weight reduction but also body-fat percentage! Watch the digits drop!

- **Easy meal preparation!**

  If I can prepare these dishes then anyone can as I can't really cook! It literally takes minutes to prepare the dishes and they can be eaten to suit you and your family's meal times.

- **Fits easily into any schedule or lifestyle!**

  All of the meals and food can be pre-prepared and stored so you can take it wherever you go. No embarrassing weird shakes or concoctions that let everyone know in your workplace that you're dieting!

- **You still can live and have a social life!**

  This is the reason we created the 7 Day Bomb. A diet where you can't go out or socialize for months on end is setup to fail. The 7 Day Bomb allows you this luxury.

I just want to close the introduction to this book by saying well done for taking action and buying this book and reading it! There is a quote that says "the first step towards getting somewhere is to decide that you are not going to stay where you are". You have made a decision already in your head, then you bought this book – keep that momentum going. Schedule a start date for your diet within 5 minutes of finishing this book and you can only succeed.

Below is a quote that helped me take action when I first stood butt naked in front of our bathroom mirror a few years ago – and stood before me was a fat disgusting man who I hardly recognized as myself. I took responsibility of what goes into my mouth and today – I finally like the look of that guy in the mirror.

"The best years of your life are the ones in which you decide your problems are your own. You do not blame them on your mother, the ecology, or the president. You realize that you control your own destiny" **Albert Ellis**

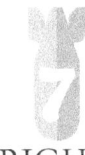

THE RIGHT WAY

"My doctor told me to stop having intimate dinners for four. Unless there are three other people." **Orson Welles**

With all the success of the 7 Day Bomb there is nothing better than receiving emails from people from all over the world telling me of their success and how the 7 Day Bomb has transformed their lives. Then there are the few emails from a few select 'haters' who say that these sorts of diets are bad for your health.

Firstly let me say this: if you are about to use the 7 Day Bomb then I encourage you to pop along and see your doctor. Show him what you are planning to do. If you know you have a medical condition then it makes sense to let your doc know beforehand. I also encourage you to read **Appendix A** (health disclaimer) before beginning the 7 Day Bomb. A copy of this is also available on the website and you can request a copy of this from us at any time (please use the contact details on the website www.7daybomb.com).

Now let's deal with these diet haters. Any diet, whether it's old or new will always attract the naysayers. Tell your friends you are about to try a new diet and you will always get one person who will say something negative or try to get you not to do it. I don't know what their reasons are; some I guess just don't want you to lose that weight as that might make them look even fatter! I totally understand people's genuine concern for others who want to lose weight and will go on a diet. But this is how I look at it. If you want to lose weight, then you must be overweight already (whether that's just a few pounds over or morbidly obese and everything in between) and I think that's quite a reasonable assumption to make. Being overweight is not healthy. I agree also that some diets may make a sudden and drastic change to your body BUT for the better! The world is facing many epidemics right now such as the financial meltdown, global warming, poverty and the growing epidemic which is now a worldwide issue: **obesity**.

Key facts

- Worldwide obesity has nearly doubled since 1980
- In 2008, more than 1.4 billion adults, 20 and older, were overweight. Of these over 200 million men and nearly 300 million women were obese
- 35% of adults aged 20 and over were overweight in 2008, 11% were obese
- 65% of the world's population live in countries where obesity kills more people than underweight people
- More than 40 million children under the age of five were overweight in 2011
- Obesity is preventable

So looking at those facts taken directly from the World

Health Organization website I bet most people's doctors would be delighted at their patients taking 7 days off fast food, alcohol and other bad stuff and giving their heart a break!

And let's not forget those that are dying of hunger. 13.1% of the world's population is hungry right now. 16,000 children die each day from hunger-related causes according to FoodBank.org

So it really does get on my nerves when people attack others for trying to lose weight. Personally, if I were obese and facing type 2 diabetes and heart disease including the risk of heart attack and strokes, or other serious consequences such as cancer and the only way to reduce my risk of these things was to diet yet people were telling me it's dangerous to diet – I know what I would do.

So if I now stop ranting and climb down from my soapbox the key takeaway here is this: go and see your doctor and let him/her know what you are doing. If you are worried that dieting will affect your health then get the facts, do your research and make up your own mind. It's your body. Don't listen to negative naysayers.

Now I have got that out of the way – let's get down to business.

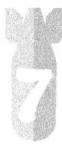

RIGHT HERE, RIGHT NOW

"Do not dwell in the past; do not dream of the future,
concentrate the mind on the present moment" **Buddha**

Now just because I have started this chapter with a quote from Buddha this means we all get defensive and judgmental. **STOP!** I am not a Buddhist and this chapter is absolutely nothing to do with Buddhism or religion. This chapter is to get you to focus on the task ahead – <u>losing 7 pounds in 7 days</u>. So please, take a minute, breathe and let go of any judgments you just had. Have they gone? Great – then let's move into this chapter which will deal with our mind and how we can ensure we have the right mindset to begin the 7 Day Bomb.

I have had many emails from people taking the 7 Day Bomb or looking to take the 7 Day Bomb and one common question is this: "What is the number one reason people fail at diets?" It's a tough question to answer because people want a simple one-line answer and also a quick fix. So after spending hours and hours researching this I have concluded it is this: I believe that to succeed at a diet consists of two key areas. They are simply **mind** and **strategy**.

I would even go as far to say it takes more effort on the mind part than the strategy. The strategy being what diet you follow and we all know there are thousands of these out there. People try them and fail, try another and fail, try another and fail – why? Because they have not got the right mindset for it. They are simply not prepared. This is why the weight loss industry is so big – new diets promise success but deep down the companies behind mass market diets know you will most likely fail and so come up with more of them. I would say it takes around 90% mind and 10% strategy. What makes the 7 Day Bomb different to all of the other diets is its 7 day approach.

ALL THAT MATTERS IS THE PRESENT

Now going back to my Buddha quote, the message here is not to live in the past, or even in the future but in the **present**. There is no such thing as the past or the future really. It does not exist. The only thing that exists is the now, right now. That's quite a profound statement to make. Think about it for a moment. Wherever you are right now reading this very sentence. Stop and think that this is RIGHT NOW. I remember going through that first year trying to lose weight. I would look back at my past failures when I attempted a diet and it depressed me. It almost said that I will most likely fail again. I then took hope about the future – I made plans for yet another diet, I told my wife that in 3 months I would be thin! The thought of the future made me momentarily happy, but it was just short lived hope that I was hanging onto. Meanwhile I was fat and unhappy. I carried on delaying the start date of the diet as my mind told me that in the future (someday) I would be thin. But because I wasn't living in the present I kept pushing the 'future' further away. I would regularly think "I failed at my diet today (as I always have done) so I will start again on Monday (future and delay)". That means your present life is unhappy. If you focus on the present ONLY and just set aside the past and set aside the future you will succeed. You don't need the past. The past does not define you. You are not the sum total of your past, your failures, your problems, your bad habits. You are a capable, unique person with so much potential. The past is just experience. Don't focus on the future either. That might sound crazy but why take your eye off the NOW? If you focus on the now you will get to the future in no time.

This thinking really helped me stick to my 7 Day Bomb attempts. Remember I was just like you, failed many times at many different diets. My past kept on telling me I couldn't do this or that. My future kept promising that everything will be ok and giving me a little bit of hope. But my present just stayed the same miserable state. Weak attempts at diets and then weight gain that left me very unhappy. The future had been promising me thinness and happiness for nearly 3 years! It wasn't until I gave up my attachment to this "happiness is in the future" lie that I realized focusing on a future dream was just delaying my weight loss. So by now I hope you can see that your past has no control of your present situation, and that the future will come whether you like it or not and you hardly have any power over it. Throwing issues that you face now into the future will just cause delay and pain. It will mean no action towards that goal in the present, therefore you will never get there – it will always be a future goal.

AWARENESS

So how do you forget the past and the future? How do we live in the present? It's quite simple, as humans and especially dieters we like to overcomplicate things. The first step is to be aware. What does that mean? It means try and watch your thoughts throughout the day. Make a mental acknowledgement when you find your mind drifting into the past. Once you start to become aware of your thoughts living/thinking in the past and the future – you can simply choose to acknowledge it and then think about the present. Bring it back to the present. The present is the actual moment you stop. Whether you're at work at a desk, in your car or maybe out walking. Our minds work at 100 miles per hour so take regular breaks in the day where you can just stop – and just look around you, feel your face with your hand, take a deep breath and focus on your breath going in and out of your body. You breathe so much in a day you never notice it. It sounds silly but it really does make your mind focus on the now. Right now as I write this I am in my office. The window looks out onto a beautiful field and then there is nothing but the sky. I have just spent a minute watching one cloud slowly drift by. My mind is not in the past, or the future – but in the present. As I sit here right now none of my worries about the future, the unknown are actually affecting me. I am alive, healthy, thin and very happy.

It will take a while for you to master the art of being aware – but if you're not watching your thoughts, you will be led in chains by your thoughts and emotions. If those thoughts are negative or based on the past or the future – whatever you're doing in the present such as dieting will go right out of the window. So being present on the 7 Day Bomb means you focus day by day, then hour by hour on that. If your mind says "I'm hungry let's eat cake" you want to be in a position to observe that thought and stop it. We will deal with some tactics on how to fight hunger later in the book. In our house now we never say "I'm starving" or "I'm hungry". We just hear those thoughts and take action to change the situation before these thoughts turn into an action such as eating cake! Naomi and I both felt really awake after learning these awareness techniques so much that it has also helped us in other areas of our lives. Below are some techniques you can follow to get started on this.

Now usually I hate cheesy acronyms but I can't deny that they have helped me remember what to do! I used a different system to Naomi; but each of them worked for us, so take a look and give it a try:

R.A.I.N

You could use these as a bit of self-therapy to stop these past negative thoughts and emotions stealing my presence and success away. So I would set 4 daily reminders in my Google Calendar that would ping me an email throughout the day and in it would be the following:

R – is to **recognize** when a strong emotion is present

A – is to **allow** or **acknowledge** that it is indeed there

I – is to **investigate** and bring self-inquiry to the body, feelings and mind – so how do you feel emotionally, physically, don't confront the emotion or try and reject it, just watch it arise and pass away

N – is to **non-identify** with what's there

This non-identification is very useful in that it helps to deflate the story and cultivates wise understanding in the recognition that the emotion is just another passing mind state and not a definition of who you are. Just like watching a movie, standing back and watching the actors play out their dramas, by non-identifying with your story and seeing it as impermanent, this will help assist in loosening your own tight grip of identification. I must admit that it takes quite a bit of courage to delve into your own mind. I know from looking at mine at first it was a right mess. We live in such a pain denying culture, especially in men. Isn't it time to begin acknowledging stress, past issues, our inner demons, insecurities and pain rather than suppressing, repressing, or all too quickly medicating it? Can we learn to view these challenges as they are instead of running away from them? Remember the key here is not to ignore these thoughts as they won't go away and at the same time don't get angry with these thoughts and try and give them more thought! Just observe them.

S.T.O.P

Naomi preferred to use this method which is less about the emotions and thoughts and more about being aware and present.

S – Stop what you are doing; put things down for a minute

T – Take a breath. Breathe normally and naturally and follow your breath coming in and out of your nose. You can even say to yourself "in" as you're breathing in and "out" as you're breathing out if that helps with concentration.

O – Observe your thoughts (don't think but observe), feelings, and emotions. You can reflect about what is on your mind and also notice that thoughts are not facts and they are not permanent. If the thought arises that you are inadequate, just notice the thought, let it be, and continue on. Notice any emotions that are there and just name them. Recent research out of UCLA says that just naming your emotions can have a calming effect. Then notice your body. Are you standing or sitting? How is your posture? Any aches or pains? Label everything as "thinking" and then return to your breathing. Watch the power melt away.

P – Proceed with something that will support you in the

moment. Whether that is talking to a friend or just rubbing your shoulders.

I'M NOT EATING THAT!

Lastly I wanted to mention your minds approach to the actual diet (if you haven't already skipped ahead to see what you can and can't eat!) Usually you would look at a diet and make judgments based on what you like and do not like. You need to stop this straight away. It's a diet – it's not meant for pleasure. If you want pleasure then think about the food you can eat on Day 8 after completing the 7 Day Bomb! Seriously – I get so many questions from people saying "What if I don't like grapefruit?" Tough! I hate grapefruit so much it nearly makes me sick. But I still eat it as I want to lose the maximum weight in the 7 days. I will talk about rules and what you can and can't do later in the book – in fact I am explicit about the rules so you shouldn't have any doubt or questions about what you can and can't do. But do not approach this diet with a "pick-n-mix" attitude or you will fail. I am telling you this now so when your mind does throw a panic later when you see the menu you can STOP it and accept that this is what it is. I know each time I swallow a piece of grapefruit, my mouth and face screw-up in reaction to the utter disgust of the taste but in my mind I see a fat naked me in the mirror! The grapefruit then almost tastes nice!

Mindfulness is a great way to approach a diet – no other diet book ever focuses on this subject but it's an essential tool to fight the fat. You may want to use a journal when you first begin and you can then see a pattern of emotions emerging. Live in the now. Most of our worries are either in the past as regret and guilt or in the future as fear and which probably won't even happen. Just focus on the now, as the now gets better you won't need the past and the future will be a thin one!

Here is a great quote I noted down in an old journal years ago which I love to read every day, so I will end this chapter with it:

"Yesterday is gone. Tomorrow has not yet come. We have only today. Let's begin" -**Mother Teresa**

DEFINE YOUR REASON

"A recent police study found that you're much more likely to get shot by a fat cop if you run" **Dennis Miller**

Having a specific reason for losing weight is going to help you immensely. If you just decide that you need to lose a few pounds, you might not! I remember when I had just got the first few revisions of the 7 Day Bomb together and we were trialing it before our holiday to Portugal. I came home from work one evening and I thought I had gone mad. Everywhere in my house were these brightly colored bikinis that Naomi had hung everywhere! Why? Because it was a great way of constantly reminding her what she was dieting for. Naomi really wanted to look good and feel good in her bikinis on the beach. I am not kidding you I even walked into the kitchen to sit down for dinner and there were two in there! One hanging by the fridge and the other hanging over our daughters treat cupboard! It was so effective.

So what's your reason? I really want you to examine your mind now and have a strong reason for this 7 day period. Below is a list of ideas which the 7 Day Bomb was originally designed for:

- Holiday
- Wedding
- Presentation at work
- Date
- Party
- Post baby weight
- Kick-starting a diet

If you are struggling to have a definitive reason for losing weight using the 7 Day Bomb then let's dig a bit deeper. If you feel like you just don't like your body, or you're not happy with your weight, or you just want your clothes to fit a bit better then I want you to think of a time where you have felt some pain associated with these things. For example, I remember after gaining weight since my wedding, friends were looking through photos from the big day and someone made a comment that I had put a few pounds on since and we laughed it off. But deep down it hurt a little so I remember the very first 7 Day Bomb I did, this was my reason, and it pushed me through the hard times. Another example from Naomi was her post baby weight. Naomi had been wearing maternity clothes for so long she wanted to try and get back into her slim dresses and skinny jeans. I remember one night finding Naomi in tears in bed because she had attempted to try almost all of her clothes on! Again this became her reason and she picked a few dresses and jeans out and kept them out as a visual to spur her on. Now any holiday or any social event will be our reason. We can't afford then to quit during our 7 Day Bomb period as we know it will impact an upcoming event. So don't just say "I want to lose weight". Make it personal. We have found the more painful the reason (or reasons) e.g. someone called you fat – the better! One of our first trial bombers, an incredible guy called Johnson from the US was morbidly obese when he contacted us to test out the 7 Day Bomb. His number one motivation was his 2 kids Jake and Corey. He had been told if he didn't lose weight then he would never make it to see his kids get married or even possibly graduate! There is no better motivation than family, especially if you have kids but think about it – the healthier you are; the happier they will be as you can be there for them. Your health does not just affect you – it affects everyone that loves you.

Once you have your reason you now need to create as many visuals and reminders of this reason as possible. I even go to the extreme length for example, before we go away on family holidays I now have random holiday photos of us all pop-up on my email via Google Calendar. So throughout the day at work I get excited and stay committed. I even have known people drive to the airport before a holiday to get pumped about it! That's commitment! But use photos, music, post-it notes, clothes or anything that will constantly remind you why you are suffering!

COMMIT

When you secretly start a diet and you screw up and fail – nobody knows and there is no pain. Because there is no pain it's easy to screw up and fail time and time again. We never ever want a person to start the 7 Day Bomb with failure on their mind. Do not start this if you are not ready. Get your mindset right – dump the junk of the past and the future and live in the present, in the now. Next – define your reason for doing this. Now I am going to ask you to commit. Commitment is a big thing but it says something- it says that you are going to give this everything you've got. I want to support each and every person that drops the 7 Day Bomb.

I now want you to go to our Facebook fan page over at www.facebook.com/7daybomb and Like us. As you will learn in the next chapter we advise you to start the 7 Day Bomb on a Friday. This is purely based on the fact that research and trials have found this is the most successful day to begin on (more on this later). Now every Thursday there will be a post on our Facebook wall that asks who is committing for the week ahead starting on the Friday. If you are seriously committed to dropping the 7 Day Bomb on your body – then like the post and make a commitment statement underneath like the following "*I am committed to dropping the 7 Day Bomb on my body this week and my reason for this is my family holiday to Portugal which is the following week*". You can put what you like but we need that commitment promise plus your reason. You have now publically made your declaration and you have also joined others who will be doing the same thing. On the following Thursday we then have a results post where we ask you for your results of how much you have lost. You are now officially a bomber!

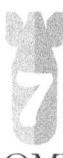

7 DAY BOMB MENU

"As a child my family's menu consisted of two choices: take it or leave it" **Buddy Hackett**

Welcome to the 7 Day Bomb menu! It isn't that bad! If you think it is bad – remember it's only for 7 days!

Day	Breakfast	Lunch	Dinner
1	1 slice of dry toast with 1 grilled tomato	Fresh fruit – as much as you like	2 hard boiled eggs mixed in a salad Grapefruit
2	Grapefruit 1 boiled egg	Grilled chicken with tomatoes	Grilled steak and salad
3	Grapefruit 1 boiled egg	Fresh fruit – as much as you like	2 grilled lamb chops and salad Grapefruit
4	1 slice of dry toast	Fresh fruit – as much as you like	2 hardboiled eggs mixed in a salad Grapefruit
5	1 slice dry toast	Fresh fruit – as much as you like	Fresh fish and salad
6	1 glass of grapefruit juice	Fresh fruit – as much as you like	Grilled chicken and carrots Grapefruit
7	Scrambled eggs with grilled tomatoes	2 poached eggs with spinach	Grilled steak and salad

I know you now have about 100 questions about the menu so I have dedicated the entire next chapter to the rules and the law of the 7 Day Bomb. Below I have added a little bit on what you can drink on the 7 Day Bomb. If it's not listed below – you can't drink it!

DRINKS

I guess the first question after reading what you can eat is what can you drink? So below are the only drinks you are allowed:

- Water
- Black coffee or tea (no sugar, sweeteners OK if you must!)
- Green tea

You can only drink grapefruit juice when it is listed above. Water is so important. If you hate the taste of water (like my wife does) then unfortunately you are going to just have to stomach it! One tip that my wife does is she drinks ice-cold water with a good squeeze of lemon juice to sweeten it up. She puts the ice in the glass, squeezes the lemon, adds the lemon and leaves it for a few minutes, and then comes back to drink it. Another tip is to ABS – Always Be Sipping!

The amount a person needs to drink to avoid getting dehydrated will vary depending on a range of factors, including their size, the temperature, and how active they are. As a guide it is recommended that we should drink at least 1.2 litres of fluid every day. This works out to be about six 200ml or eight 150ml glasses. Most people are dehydrated most of the time and with the 7 Day Bomb we need to ensure we are drinking lots of water.

My preference is to split my day into blocks of two hours. In these two hours I will drink a pint of ice cold water and a green tea. In addition to this I will have around 3 black coffees in the morning as this gives me my caffeine kick but I don't drink any coffee after 11am as it will still be running around my body when I am trying to get to sleep later in the night. One cup of coffee has 100-150mg of caffeine; a cup of green tea has only about 25mg of caffeine and bear in mind it takes around 6 hours for caffeine to travel through the body. So after my morning coffees I then switch to green teas. Green teas rock! I have green tea with lemon and it is quite nice. Green tea is made from unfermented leaves and reportedly contains the highest concentration of powerful antioxidants called polyphenols. Antioxidants are substances that fight free radicals – damaging compounds in the body that change cells, damage DNA, and even cause cell death. Many scientists believe that free radicals contribute to the ageing process as well as the development of a number of health problems, including cancer and heart disease. Antioxidants found in green tea basically neutralize these damaging free radicals.

In addition to my always be sipping habit and my green teas I also down a large glass of ice cold water when I'm hungry (as we will learn later in the book) so this also ensures that I am having plenty of water. Another little check nature has to remind me I am drinking lots is the hourly trips to the toilet! Naomi will have 2 large glasses of ice cold water before breakfast (one as soon as she wakes up and one right before breakfast). She then has 2 more before lunch plus a couple of green teas and then one directly before lunch, 2 more in the afternoon plus more green teas (as many as you can drink!) Then a glass before dinner and depending upon exercise she will have 2 more glasses before bed.

So many people do not drink enough, and when they email saying they're not losing the weight, I go through an analysis of everything that's past their lips in the past 24 hours - I immediately see why. So to ensure we understand how important water is, let's take a look at some more ways water will help shift that weight!

- **It fills you up** – did you know that often when you feel hungry, you're really just thirsty? Our mind tends to confuse hunger and thirst. One trick is to consume a large amount e.g. a pint which is ice cold so the sensation takes the brains attention away from hunger to deal with this large amount of cold fluid in the stomach.

- **It revs up your metabolism** – dehydration is your body's enemy. It slows bodily functions and metabolism. As a matter of fact, your metabolism will slow to conserve energy when you haven't had enough water to drink, as your organs can't and won't function as efficiently. Scientifically speaking, drinking water has been proven to contribute to your body's ability to burn calories. Your body needs an adequate amount of water to properly function, especially during exercise, and dehydration prohibits the fat-burning process.

- **Flushes out the bad stuff** – water flushes toxins from your body's system, including those produced during exercise. It aids in keeping your joints lubricated – very important for both daily functions and in preventing your body from injury during exercise. The body is made up of 50 – 65% of water so ensure you're topped up!

NO SUGAR!

Absolutely no sugar. I struggled with this but it's just 7 days and there are other options such as having lemon juice in your water and tea! People ask if they can use sweeteners and I still think "come on its just 7 days!" If you must have something sweet in your tea and coffees then go ahead and use sweetener. I would advise only use the sweeteners in the tablet form and not the loose powder form (as you can't control the amount you shovel in!) I would also limit the sweeteners to 4 per day. So why am I so nervous about artificial sweeteners? Well there has been some research done which looks at the effect artificial sweeteners have on the body. Scientists have found that when the body tastes a sweet taste it prepares the stomach and the acids and digestion process for something sweet and high in calories. When nothing high in calories arrives in the stomach it will then send a signal to the brain to say "I'm hungry". So I don't want you getting that hunger feeling especially when you will be close to hungry anyway!

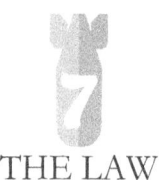

THE LAW

"Taste cannot be controlled by law" **Thomas Jefferson**

What an opening quote! Taste <u>will be</u> controlled by the law in this chapter! The true success of the 7 Day Bomb is to live within the law. The law is here to protect you from the ways of failure. Every law here has been either learnt the hard way or exists from experience whether practical or scientific. Now you may not always stick to the speed limit when you drive, you may be late occasionally paying your taxes, but please obey the 7 Day Bomb law!

I have found that you can tell people "here is the only food and drink you consume for one week on this plan" and they still come back and ask can they eat this or that! So my rule of thumb is this – <u>if it isn't on the menu, you can't have it.</u>

<u>THE LAW</u>

<u>PUNISHMENT – If you choose to break the law, you get to keep the weight!</u>

1. Stick to the plan.

2. Stick to the plan!!!
3. Do not swap meals around to suit you. Leave the meals where they are.
4. Do not substitute anything. If you do not like anything then try and eat it (even if you wash it down with water). If you physically cannot eat it then you go without but please try. ***NOTE:** There are three exceptions only – see below.
5. No eating between meals. Eat only what is shown at the specific time period e.g. breakfast, lunch, dinner.
6. No snacking
7. No sauces or garnishes – only a squeeze of lemon allowed
8. No alcohol
9. Only drinks allowed are water, black tea/coffee, green tea – no fizzy drinks, no diet drinks or juices allowed (even sugar free juices)

People FAIL at this plan because they do not stick to the plan. Stick to the plan and you cannot go wrong. It's just 7 days people! So please don't start going through the menu with a pen saying "I don't like that or this". If it was a month long plan then fair enough it would be different but this is 7 measly days! My wife and I both HATE grapefruit with a passion. It literally makes our faces screw up in disgust but we throw it in our mouths and wash it down with water. Why? Because we want to lose 7 pounds in 7 days! So please stick to the plan! 7 pounds is some serious weight loss! It's a belt buckle down, fitting back into those jeans, a better look in the mirror and a happier you!

THREE EXCEPTIONS

So there has to be a little room for some of the stuff so here are the ONLY three exceptions:

1. **Vegetarian**: Naturally you can swap the meat dishes for an alternative replacement such as Quorn
2. **Fish**: If you can't handle anything nautical then replace with chicken.
3. **Grapefruit**: If you can't stomach grapefruit (even after trying to down small pieces with water!) then go and get pink grapefruit. It's a little sweeter and less bitter.

For any other questions then please visit our Facebook page www.facebook.com/7daybomb where we will have regular Q&A sessions. Just look out for the Q&A posts and post your question in the comments.

1. **Stick to the plan**

2. **If you can't eat it – go without**

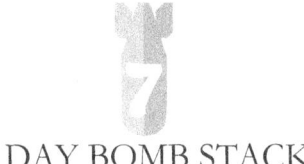

7 DAY BOMB STACK

"I keep trying to lose weight… but it keeps finding me"

USING THE 7 DAY BOMB AS AN ONGOING DIET

So you want to use the 7 Day Bomb as an ongoing diet as opposed to the 7 day period? That's fine. As mentioned before the 7 Day Bomb was never designed for following for more than the 7 days. If someone did do this then they would find that their body would go into starvation mode and this would prevent the body shedding any more weight – so please read carefully if you plan to use the 7 Day Bomb as an ongoing diet.

WARNING!

Because you lose so much weight in one week of the 7 Day Bomb your body by the end of the week will be getting ready to go into starvation mode. This is the body's way of preserving as much fat as possible as it thinks you're not going to eat for a while. So as you can imagine if you keep on the 7 Day Bomb into week two then you will suffer as you will be hungry, you won't be eating much and you won't lose weight! Some people don't listen and email saying they lost nothing in week two! Don't do it!

There is a way and it's called…

7 DAY BOMB STACK

The 7 day Bomb Stack uses the 7 Day Bomb 7 day plan over a period of 3 -6 months or however long you need it to get to your healthy weight. So if you have a lot to lose then you can grab yourself a calendar and work out when you do the 7 Day Bomb like this. Using a 10 week stack for example:

WEEK 1 - 7 Day Bomb
WEEK 2 - Swing
WEEK 3 - 7 Day Bomb
WEEK 4 - Swing
WEEK 5 - Swing
WEEK 6 - 7 Day Bomb
WEEK 7 - Swing
WEEK 8 - 7 Day Bomb
WEEK 9 – Swing
WEEK 10 - Swing
Then repeat…

SWING

So **swing** is our term for what you eat in the weeks between the 7 Day Bomb stacks.

Swing is based on the premise of the following core points:

1. Core diet based on slow-carbohydrate
2. Avoid processed foods

3. Avoid variety – this makes it easy to stick to
4. One cheat day per week (to bring the body out of starvation mode)

I've not put a meal plan in here on purpose. A strict meal plan is only for a short term stint such as the 7 Day Bomb – but when you are not doing a hardcore regime like the 7 Day Bomb you must select some dishes that at least satisfy you. So during the swing weeks I would recommend you selecting some meals from hundreds of good free menu sites such as Linda's Low Carb Menu & Recipes website which is here www.genaw.com/lowcarb

SLOW-CARB DIET FOOD PLAN

Slow-Carb Diet – what to eat – 6 days a week + breakfast on "cheat day"

- <u>Eat the same few meals over and over again</u>. Pick three or four meals and repeat them. Water, unsweetened tea / coffee.
- <u>Proteins</u> – as much as you like – eggs, chicken breast or thigh, beef, fish, pork. Eat at least 20 grams of protein per meal.
- <u>Legumes</u> – as much as you like – lentils, black beans, pinto beans, red beans, soy beans
- <u>Vegetables</u> – as much as you like - spinach, broccoli, cauliflower, other cruciferous vegetables, sauerkraut, kimchee, asparagus, peas, green beans. There's no need to limit yourself to these vegetables, although the more variety you attempt the more likely you are to quit as this makes the diet more complicated.
- <u>Tomatoes and avocadoes are allowed</u>.
- <u>Butter is fine</u>. Cottage cheese is also

acceptable.

- <u>Oils</u> - Olive oil, grape seed oil and macadamia oil, as well as nuts as a source of fat, are preferred.
- Canned foods are fine.
- Drink plenty of water.
- Timing: Make sure you have your first meal within an hour of waking (preferably within ½ hour), and have meals approximately 4 hours apart.

Slow-Carb Diet – foods to avoid – 6 days a week + breakfast on "cheat day"

- <u>Avoid "white" carbohydrates</u>. No bread, rice (including brown), whole grains, cereal including processed oats, potatoes, pasta, tortillas, and fried food with breading. Cauliflower is ok.
- <u>Don't drink calories</u>. Do not drink milk (including soy milk), normal soft drinks, or fruit juice. Limit soft drinks to no more than 16 ounces per day, as the aspartame can stimulate weight gain (as I discussed earlier about artificial sweeteners). No alcohol.
- <u>Don't eat fruit or fructose</u>.
- <u>No dairy</u>
- <u>Avoid refined soy products</u>, if possible, including soy milk.
- <u>Don't deep fry foods</u> – stir fry is okay.
- <u>Be careful with "domino foods"</u> – nuts, chickpeas, hummus, peanuts, macadamias. They are very easy to overeat and prone to portion abuse. A few almonds (5-10) are fine.
- <u>Limit consumption of artificial and natural</u>

sugar substitutes, they can stall weight loss.

Slow-Carb Diet – what to eat – 1 "cheat day" a week

- Take one day off a week, preferably a weekend when you will have time off and relax with a few treats. Don't go crazy as some people would! I always go for a long morning walk after breakfast on a cheat day, and then I might have a chocolate bar with a cup of tea, a burger for lunch and then maybe a pack of crisps in the afternoon. For tea I might have a takeaway but nothing of multiple portions. Remember to just enjoy foods you have missed. The next day I would then think about exercise, walking etc

- Drink plenty of water – so important to keep the body flushed. Remember – it's not about going mental here – we are just getting the calorie intake to spike so your body can pull out of starvation mode.

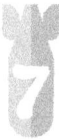

TIPS, TRICKS & ADVICE

*"Oh you want to lose 3 pounds for bikini season? I had to eat
3 raw carrots for lunch just to squeeze back into my fat jeans!"*
Naomi found this on a birthday card

I want to share with you here some practical tips that
Naomi and I picked up along the way; not only what we
found helped during the 7 Day Bomb but also in our 1,000
years of dieting (or so it feels like it). What's different here
to the many other diet books is we promise no secrets or
miracles. Just simple stuff that works. So again with
anything, give it a try and see what works for you.

STOP LOOKING AHEAD

I remember starting a new diet – the excitement and
belief that "this is the one" really made me feel almost
thinner! But this feeling soon vanished away along with
any weight loss plan! I would usually read up on the diet,
set a date (always in the future) and then have what I called
a last treat weekend where I would probably gain an extra
6 pounds which never helps does it! I would then sit down
on day one and always be thinking ahead. What can I eat
tomorrow and the day after and before I knew it my mind
was weighed down (excuse the pun) with worry and
depression at how long I had to go.

So my advice here is focus on the day you're on and that's it. Forget the rest. Stop saying "oh I wish it was Wednesday as we can have roast chicken on Wednesday". See the day through. One day at a time. Perfect each day and before you know it you will be at the end of day 7 and 7 pounds lighter. Remember what 7 pounds is! It's a small dog, a new born baby, a big fish! It's a lot! For me it meant new shirts, a new belt, old fashionable clothes that I could start wearing again. 7 pounds is awesome!

FRESH FRUIT & VEG

This tip comes from Naomi. As there is quite a bit of fruit and vegetables on this 7 day plan Naomi always likes it to be fresh. So rather than going out the day before you start and buying everything, space it out to a few days at a time. This way you can ensure your fruit and vegetables are fresh.

PRESENTATION

It's easy when you have fruit for lunch to eat an apple, then peel a banana and then pick a few grapes and then you're done. It doesn't feel like you have had a lunch, just a few snacks. So prepare your fruit salad like you have just been served at a health farm, or a 5 star restaurant on a cruise ship. Take your fruit to work but go and spend 5 minutes preparing it. Chop the fruit so it's a salad, squeeze orange juice from your chopped oranges over the top and then stick it all in a bowl. This way it feels like a meal and not just fruit as your irrational hungry mind might be labeling the situation as!

HUNGER PAIN

Firstly it is not pain but I know it can feel like that when you're hungry! During the 7 Day Bomb the only real time you will feel hungry is about 2 hours before you are due to eat next. So firstly, let's put this into perspective – it's only 2 hours! Secondly, go back to our mindfulness teachings earlier in this book – try and stop yourself and watch, feel the emotion of hunger arise. Watch out for the little voice that wants you to eat. This voice will try and reason with you that eating something naughty is going to help and that it won't be that bad. Don't ruin your week – stop and listen to that thought. Then I want you to mentally acknowledge this bully inside your head. Next step is to stop whatever it is you are doing and go to the fridge and pull out chilled water. Fill up a pint glass and drop in three or 4 chunks of ice. Let the ice chill the water for 3 minutes and then down the glass of water in one go. The amount of water will fill your stomach and satisfy that feeling and the coldness of it will also divert the minds attention from getting you to eat into warming your body core up. Then remind yourself that it's only a few hours until your next meal and get on with the struggle. Remind yourself why you are doing this – pull out an image, or think of that reason and get that motivation back. Think about what weight you have lost so far – say "I'm not going to ruin this week".

STOP RUSHING

In our house there are two types of mornings. The first is what I like. It's a chilled out morning, plenty of time for talking, take a shower, eat, pick an outfit for the day, check the email, weather and news and then set off with plenty of time to go. Or there is the second type – completey manic where any agenda, breakfast, shower and ironed clothes go out the window. If your morning falls into the latter of these that I have described then I really want to encourage you to make a real effort during the 7 Day Bomb to get up a little earlier and allow yourself time to prepare for the day. Naomi is great in that she will get food and things ready the evening before which means we just grab what we need. But one of the biggest failures in the 7 Day Bomb is from people telling me they haven't had time to eat properly. If that's the case then you don't have time to lose weight and you don't have time for your own health. I have known some people so dedicated to the 7 Day Bomb that they have booked a week off work to fully focus on the plan. It makes sense also to pick a week where you are able to say no to any social events or occasions where you will either be expected to eat any offered food or where you might be placed into temptation.

LEMON IS YOUR FRIEND

Lemon juice can transform your salads and even your water and green teas into a delicious dish.

PINT OF WATER BEFORE A MEAL

A pint or large glass of ice cold water before you start to eat will help you get that full and satisfied feeling. It isn't just a feeling for you but your body will also be satisfied and will stop with the hunger signals all the time.

GET A DIET BUDDY

I bet there will be hundreds of people that want to join you for 7 days to lose 7 pound. So text a few buddies to see if they want to join you on this life changing journey.

WATCH OUT FOR BUMBPS IN THE ROAD

During your week you will face difficult and stressful situations as you do in any normal week in life. Trouble at work, stress about debt, a breakup or some bad news. But turn that around – use that as a catalyst to spur you on, use the 7 Day Bomb as one thing you will focus on and use it to get you to the end of that week. We must try; and I know it's hard, to stop using bad news to derail every diet attempt. Unfortunately a week without bad news and issues isn't going to happen so we need to be aware of this. I remember one tip I used to do is say to myself each day "something will happen today that I am not going to be happy about, but when it does come up I am ready". Low and behold 3pm that day I would get some bad news or a situation would come up that wasn't very pretty and I was able to say "there it is" and catch it. There is immense power in being able to do that and it transformed over time the way I deal with crap that crops up! Try it!

JOIN IN WITH OTHER BOMBERS

Join in with other bombers from around the world on our Facebook.com/7daybomb fan page. We will also be holding Q&A sessions and also giving you the chance to share your experiences and tips.

POWER OF SAYING "NO"

Last piece of advice is from a quote that I heard Russell Simmons (music tycoon) say "**not doing what you feel like doing is freedom**". I love that quote – because once you have the gift and power of saying no to that cake at that party, that biscuit at work, those chocolates at home means you are free from the power of temptation that it had over you. Celebrate that – that is power, self-control and strength.

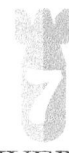

THE SHIVER SYSTEM

"Nothing burns like the cold" **George RR Martin**

I can recall Naomi ordering this weird thick fitness outfit some years back that I named a sweat-suit. She said it was a triple insulated costume that would increase her body's temperature and make her sweat, meaning she would burn calories. But I believe it's the other way round: I believe that exposing the body to cold can be an effective spur for losing weight.

I read about a US Olympic swimmer called Michael Phelps who when training would consume 12,000 calories per day, bearing in mind the average male should consume around 2,500 per day! I then read about a guy called Ray Cronise a NASA material scientist who had also read about Michael Phelps and has taken on this study into how the cold can assist weight-loss.

It's quite simple: if you expose your body to the cold, whether you immerse yourself in a bath of cold water or go for a walk in a vest and shorts in a snow-storm your body is going to be burning a huge amount of calories in two ways. Firstly, your body will burn extra calories to maintain your body's core temperature of 37 degrees and it will also have energy sucked out of the body via the cold.

Ray Cronise was carrying an extra few pounds so as part of his research he put himself through some tests. So one Autumn Ray took cool showers, slept without any duvet, and took long walks wearing just light clothing. In six weeks Ray shed 12kg! He tripled his weight-loss rate without changing his calorie-restricted diet.

From Ray's experiment and incredible results an entire industry has been setup to provide solutions to people who want to shed weight using the cold. Timothy Ferriss in his book *The 4-Hour Body* talks about taking ice baths! There are also sports outfits like my wife's sweat-suit that have adapted pockets where you can put ice packs into! But it's important not to get carried away here – the cold is not nice and if you get it wrong you could do quite a bit of harm.

SENSIBLE SHIVERING

I was very inspired by all of this research and so decided to conduct my own experiment with the cold alongside the 7 Day Bomb and luckily for me it was the middle of winter here in the UK. Rather than taking ice baths and living in an igloo in my garden when it snowed I went for a more sensible shiver system and want to share this with you. But before I dive into some tips on how I used the power of the cold to lose an extra few pounds I want to state that this is not part of the 7 Day Bomb – even if you do not do this you will still lose 7 pounds. This will help you take a bit extra off.

Shiver Walks
Take 30 minute walks in the cold wearing shorts and a t-shirt. But please cover up your head, ears and hands. These areas will get damaged by the cold if you do not

protect them. Your legs, arms and core will be exposed enough to the cold that they will begin working overtime to regulate the heat.

Ice Drinks

Replace every drink with ice cold water. Ensure the water is chilled and fill a glass with a lot of ice. Let the ice sit in the water so the temperature lowers and then drink it in one go. Overloading the core of the body with this amount of ice cold water will significantly lower the body's core temperature and it will again burn calories in warming it back up. Try and do this once an hour.

Gradual Cold Baths

So remember we are not trying to put our bodies into the extremes of cold, but just get a little cooler. Start off with a lukewarm bath that you could slip into quite easily. Then slowly add cold to the water, your body can adapt without the uncomfortable suddenness and get it to a point where you feel cold. Try and then lie there for 10 minutes submerged with just your head out of the water.

Cold Opportunities

There are also lots of opportunities to get cold throughout your day. So I would leave my coat at home, I would drive with the windows down, open my office window and I once put the air conditioning on which annoyed other co-workers! You can also sleep without a duvet or sleep with a thinner sheet. Leave the heating off, open a window at night time when you sleep and spend more time outside in the cold.

So I did the above shiver system the same week as the 7 Day Bomb and from the initial tests that I did I would usually lose an extra 3 pound on top of my 7 pound lost just doing the 7 Day Bomb. The science is still out on the effects of the cold on weight loss but the results speak for themselves.

There's no excuse now for when the weather gets cold. Even in the warm summer months, if you rise early enough you can still grab the cool morning air that will cause you to shiver. Embrace this part of nature that you would normally wrap up against and lose an extra few pounds.

MOTHER NATURE'S GYM

"I have two doctors, my left leg and my right" **G.M. Trevelyan**

People honestly think if you buy all the accessories and have all the gear that it will be a doddle. How many brand new bikes are rusting away in sheds and garages around the world? How many gym membership direct debits are slipping out of peoples bank accounts yet they can't even locate their membership card? How many weight benches are being used as clothes horses? It's over the top, almost a distraction technique to delay starting a diet. You don't need anything!

As long as you have to two legs and you are able to physically walk then you have everything you need. Mother Nature's gym is awesome. Firstly there is no contracts to sign, no induction and it has the largest variety of equipment in the world! It also has the freshest air! Ok if you still don't know what I am on about I am talking about getting outside and walking once a day!

You don't need to go running, jogging, sprinting, cross-country or any other fast-paced sport. You don't need to go to any special classes – exercise can just be walking for 30 minutes per day. Simple as that. Since you are allocating 7 days to this you might as well throw in 30 minutes walking. If you don't walk at the moment and you don't do any physical exercise then 30 minutes walking for 7 days will do you the world of good and it will shift a few more extra pounds.

I personally love walking and will use walking as a way to meditate and a way to start my day. I love getting out before everyone else has risen, having the entire countryside to myself (or so it feels this way). I love the cold morning air as I can feel it all the way down into my lungs. No gym could give this clear pure air. I try not to think of anything as I walk, I just take in everything, become aware, touch the stone walls and contemplate how old they are, feel the wet grass and the damp cool trees as I walk past them. I might stop to listen to the pure sound of water trickling in a stream or lock by the canal. Any thoughts that come invading this space I simply label as "thinking" and return to be fully awake. I look up at the clouds, watching them as they move by – how often do we go about for weeks, months maybe years not ever stopping and admiring the clouds and sky above us. I'm not getting all spiritual on you here but try this. Go outside for 30 minutes, go deep into the country and experience this world! Don't drag all your worries with you though!

I also return to my walk at the end of the day – I try and time it so I can find a nice spot to witness the sun go down. I love seeing the sky go from bright to a purple, pink orange and red. It's a great time to just be grateful for being alive and having the family I have. The best thing while doing all of this – I am burning calories and improving my metabolism.

METABOLISM

Metabolism describes all the chemical processes that go on continuously inside the body to keep you alive and your organs functioning normally, such as breathing, repairing cells and digesting food. These chemical processes require energy. The minimum amount of energy your body requires to carry out these chemical processes is called the basal metabolic rate (BMR). Your BMR accounts for anything between 40% and 70% of your body's daily energy requirements depending on your age and lifestyle. A 'slow metabolism' is more accurately described as a low BMR. Funnily enough research has also found that people with a 'high metabolism' are just more physically active than others! So here is a real calling for you to begin walking each day.

GREAT WAY TO GET INTO FITNESS

Walking is the best way to get into fitness. You can't just suddenly start running if you currently do no exercise. If you do I can guarantee you won't even be able to walk the following day! So we need to start slowly and then add a bit here and a bit there. So 30 minutes walking a day is a great start – your legs will slowly get stronger, your lungs will be able to cope with the new demand you put on your body but it's not too much too soon that your muscles, joints and bones ache.

GET STARTED

So the first thing is to decide you're going to walk 30 minutes per day. There is an eastern saying that "everything exists on the tip of a wish". So decide in your mind first and then take action. Don't plan or schedule a start date in – get up now, get your shoes on and walk for 15 minutes. Stop, - turn around and come home! Seriously! Promise yourself for the next 7 days at least while you're doing the 7 Day Bomb you will get outside for 30 minutes walking whatever happens, whatever the weather. Even if it's literally around your block.

Enjoy it! Don't see it as I have to do 30 minutes – enjoy it, walk somewhere like up to a high point in the city or go out into the countryside that overlooks a lake or somewhere where you can feel like you're the only person in the world – nobody else around. It can be easy to get bored of a walk so change your route. I have about 5 regular routes I do – some I drive to others I can trek from my house to them. One tip is try and get up early in the morning and do your walk as it's out the way then – or if you are really committed then go for two walks, one in the morning and one in the evening. Remember – you don't need any gear – just comfortable shoes and a smile. Can you walk the kids to school instead of taking the car? Or walk to work? Get off a stop earlier? Go up and down the stairs at home twice every time you use them!

Let's take a look at what a person weighing 60kg can lose on one 30 minute walk:

- Strolling (2mph): 75 calories
- Walking (3mph): 99 calories
- Fast walking (4mph): 150 calories

When I started walking many years ago I set myself weekend walks as part of my plan which meant that I would walk for 6 days and on the 7th day I would go to somewhere like a National Park or famous walk with amazing views such as the Malvern Hills here in England. So use exercise as a treat also for a great day out with the family.

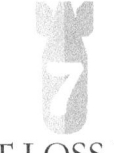

WEIGHT LOSS WISDOM

"You're not going to get the butt you want by sitting on it" **Scott Barlow**

What has been really nice about the journey of creating the 7 Day Bomb is the people who we have met whose lives have been touched in some way by the result of them losing weight following our plan. We literally receive emails from all over the world and we read and respond to each one. I have also noticed the amount of people who go onto ask for my advice on other areas of their lives.

One major point of any diet is that weight loss without lifestyle change is never permanent. You gained the weight not because you ate one meal that was different to what you normally ate; it's because of a repeated lifestyle choice. So people always ask me, what's next? Well after you have lost the first 7 pounds the biggest issue is how you keep it off. There is only one answer: **change your lifestyle**. If you don't want to change your lifestyle (for the better) then accept that you will be overweight for life. But don't waste your life by denying lifestyle change and being unhappy on a pointless diet. It's a crazy circle of depression!

Although this book is not about lifestyle change I am going to start doing some weekly blog posts on different areas of your life and how you can start to change these – you can find these on the 7 Day Bomb website (www.7daybomb.com). But to begin with I have selected 5 topics below which is real advice I have given readers in response to their questions. I hope you will find it useful as you embark on the 7 Day Bomb plan and also consider a lifestyle change.

Don't forget to visit the blog to read more.

THE HABIT OF STARTING

There are good and bad habits.

Good habits are hard to start and bad habits are hard to stop.

But what habits have in common is that if we do them often enough, they will form (and the opposite works well for stopping bad habits).

But when we start a new habit we usually focus on the quality or quantity rather than on how often we do it at first. For example, I have just started writing and my goal is to write 3,000 words each day. When I first began my mind was focused on the amount of 3,000 words per day. But really my habit should have been focused on just starting to write each day for say the first 4 weeks. Get me in a routine of waking up early, grabbing a coffee and sitting at my desk and just writing. After I do 30 days of this I can then step up the habit to writing daily and writing 3,000 words.

The key to forming a habit is starting each day.

Nothing else.

So let's look at what we mean by starting. If you want to try to form the habit of meditation, just get your butt on the cushion each day. If you want to form the habit of running, just lace up your trainers and get out the door and run. If you want to form the habit of writing, just sit down, close everything else on your laptop, and begin typing.

Form the habit of starting, and you'll get good at forming habits.

So now you have formed the habit of starting – what happens when you wake up and don't feel like doing meditation or running or writing?

Well I would first take a look at why you don't feel like starting. It's usually for one or both of these reasons:

1. You are comfortable with what you're doing, and the habit is less comfortable. For example, its comfortable reading the 7 Day Bomb book, but it's not comfortable going for a walk at 0700am in the cold. We cling to the comfortable.
2. It's too difficult to get started – to do the habit, you have to get a bunch of equipment out your garage, or drive to the gym, or go get a bunch of ingredients etc.

So these are the two main reasons but do you know what? They are essentially the same. So the solution is to make it easier and more comfortable to do the habit, and easier to get started. Here are some pointers:

- Focus on the smallest thing – just getting started.

You don't have to do even 5 minutes of walking for example – just start. That's so easy it's hard to say no!

- Prepare everything you need to get started earlier. So if you need some equipment, get it ready well before you have to start, like the evening before, or in the morning if you have to do it in the afternoon, or at least an hour before. Then when it's time to start, there is no barrier.

- Make the habit something you can do where you are, instead of having to drive there

- If you have to drive or walk somewhere, have someone meet you there. Then you're less likely to stay at home (or at work), and more likely to go – and going there is the same thing as getting started. This works because you're making it less comfortable to not start – the idea of leaving a friend waiting for you at the gym or park is not a comfortable one.

- Tell people you're going to do the habit of starting your habit every day for 30 days. Having this kind of accountability motivates you to get started, and makes it less comfortable not to start.

- Start with the easiest version of the habit, so that it's easy to start. For example, if you want to start yoga, don't try the most difficult poses but instead an easy series of moves.

Make it as easy as possible to start, and hard not to start. Tell yourself that all you have to do is lace up your trainers and get out the door, and you'll have a hard time saying no. Once you've started, you'll feel good and probably want to continue (though that's not a necessity).

The start is a sunrise: a moment of brilliance that signals something joyful has arrived. Learn to love that moment of brilliance, and your habit troubles fade like the night.

My next bit of wisdom for you is:

PRACTICAL TIPS TO PRACTICE BEING PRESENT

Before carrying on, stop. Listen to your breath for one cycle – in and then out. Good – that's present right there. How often do we breathe in and out each day that we notice?

I talked about being present earlier in the book and wanted to provide some more pointers on this:

1. **Pay Attention** – When you have idle time at a traffic light or in a queue at the supermarket, for example, pay attention. Instead of letting your mind run ahead of you thinking about the route to your destination and possible traffic delays or the list of errands that have to be completed after the shopping run, take a moment to pay attention. Turn off the radio in the car, roll down the windows and witness the traffic gong by, the jogger getting his morning run, the trees dancing in the wind, listen to the birds chirp, the rustling of the leaves. You only have to do it for a few moments, but it's a good start.

2. **Observe** – Next time you're in a meeting, observe what is going on. It's a bit more than paying attention in duration. Paying attention is on a trigger basis. Observation is like watching a movie on a

screen. Watch the players in action. Watch the body language. Listen for intonations. Do not speak. This can be a very powerful tool as you sit and take in everything that is playing out. You have nothing at stake in the grand scheme of things, but watch as you are able to respond perfectly when questioned. You will be surprised.

3. **Breathe** – When you're ready to go beyond moments and minutes, try paying attention to your breath before you drift off to sleep. Before you drift off to sleep, spend 15 minutes paying attention to the rise and fall of your belly. If you feel yourself drifting off to sleep, or notice that your mind has wondered, gently bring it back to your belly. You could even put a book on it and watch it rise and fall.

4. **Meditate** – You can now begin to establish a sitting practice. It is the practice of sitting still for about 30 minutes in silence. Let your thoughts go. When you realize that your mind is chasing your thoughts, bring it back to your breath. Just be still. Nothing to do or think about. Nothing to ponder, just be.

You can practice being present from the bottom of the list to the top also, but I find that it's easy to go with small steps. Soon, you will begin to be aware in what you are actively doing. If you are cooking, don't think about what comes next, pay attention to what you are chopping now. When you are present, your life energy is infused into all that you do, from writing code for your website, to singing a lullaby to your child, to having dinner. Give it a try – it's amazing what you have been missing!

My next bit of wisdom for you is:

GET OFF YOUR BUTT! 16 WAYS TO GET MOTIVATED

Thinking about starting a new challenge like losing weight can be scary and seem almost impossible.

But it's not hopeless: with some small steps, baby ones in fact, you can get started down the road to positive change.

I know when I get ill or have some bad news or just a stressful day we can easily fall out of positivity and give up on our diets or exercise. It even seems harder to restart! But fear not as I have been there (a few thousand times) and so here are some ways that helped me:

1. **One Goal** – go back to one goal. Whenever I've been in a slump, I've discovered that it's often because I have too much going on in my life. I'm trying to do too much. And it zaps my energy and motivation. It's probably the most common mistake that people make: they try to take on too much, try to accomplish too many goals at once. You cannot maintain energy and focus (the two most important things in accomplishing a goal) if you are trying to do two or more goals at once. It's not possible – I've tried it many times. You have to choose one goal, for now, and focus on it completely. I know, that's hard. Still, I speak from experience. You can always do your other goals when you've accomplished your One Goal – **Lose 7 Pounds in 7 Days!**
2. **Find Inspiration** – Inspiration, for me, comes from others who have achieved what I want to achieve, or who are currently doing it. I read other blogs, books, magazines. I Google my goal, and read success

stories. Look at our Facebook fan page for before and after photos – truly inspiring!

3. **Get Excited** – This sounds obvious, but most people don't think about it much: if you want to break out of a slump, get yourself excited about a goal. But how can you do that when you don't feel motivated? Well, it starts with inspiration from others (see above), but you have to take that excitement and build on it. For me, I've learned that by talking to my wife about it, and to others, and reading as much about it as possible, and visualizing what it would be like to be successful (seeing the benefits of the goal in my head), I get excited about a goal. Once I've done that, it's just a matter of carrying that energy forward and keeping it going.

4. **Build Anticipation** – This will sound hard, and many people will skip this tip. But it really works. If you find inspiration and want to do a goal, don't start right away. Many of us will get excited and want to start today. That's a mistake. Set a date in the future – a week or two, or even a month - and make that your Start Date. Mark it on the calendar. Get excited about that date. Make it the most important date in your life! In the meantime, start writing out a plan. And do some of the steps below. Because by delaying your start, you are building anticipation, and increasing your focus and energy for your goal.

5. **Post Your Goal** – Print out your goal in big words. Make your goal just a few words long, like a mantra ("exercise 15 minutes daily"), and post it up on your wall or fridge. Post it at home and work. Put it on your desktop and screensaver; post it on Facebook and Twitter! You want to have big reminders about your goal, to keep your focus and keep your

excitement going.

6. **Commit Publically** – None of us like to look bad in front of others. We will go the extra mile to do something we've said publically. For example, when I announced my engagement to my wife Naomi, I had to go through with that (joke!) But seriously a group message on Facebook to a select few friends or change your Facebook status to everyone and ask them for their support.

7. **Think About It Daily** – If you think about your goal every day, it is much more likely to become true. To this end, posting the goal on your wall or computer desktop (as mentioned above) helps a lot. Sending yourself daily reminders via Google Calendar also helps. And so if you can commit to doing one small thing to further your goal (even 5 minutes) every single day, your goal will almost certainly come true.

8. **Get Support** – It's hard facing something alone. Find a friend who would like to lose weight, say would you like to lose 7 pounds in 7 days with me? When I first started out walking I joined an online forum where I could meet other likeminded ramblers and learn about routes etc. I also had the support from my wife and friends.

9. **Realize That There's An Ebb & Flow** – Motivation is not a constant thing that is always there for you. It comes and goes, and comes and goes again, like the tide. But realize that while it may go away, it doesn't do so permanently. It will come back. Just stick it out and wait for that motivation to come back. In the meantime, read about your goal (see below), ask for help (see below), and do some of the other things listed here until your motivation comes back.

10. **Stick With It** – Whatever you do, don't give up. Even if you aren't feeling any motivation today, or this week, don't give up. Again, that motivation will come back. Think of your goal as a long journey, and your slump is just a little bump in the road. You can't give up with every little bump. Stay with it for the long term, ride out the ebbs and surf on the flows, and you'll get there.

11. **Start Small. Really Small** – If you are having a hard time getting started, it may be because you're thinking too big. If you want to exercise, for example, you may be thinking that you have to do these intense workouts 5 days a week. No – instead, do small, tiny, baby steps. Just do 2 minutes of exercise. I know, that sounds wimpy. But it works. Commit to 2 minutes of exercise for one week. You may want to do more, but just stick to 2 minutes. It's so easy, you can't fail. Do it at the same time every day. Just some crunches, 2 pushups, and some jogging on the spot. Once you've done 2 minutes a day for a week, increase it to 5, and stick with that for a week. In a month, you'll be doing 15-20. Want to wake up early? Don't think about waking at 5am. Instead, think about waking 10 minutes earlier for a week. That's all. Once you've done that, wake 10 minutes earlier than that. Baby steps.

12. **Build On Small Successes** – Again, if you start small for a week, you're going to be successful. You can't fail if you start with something ridiculously easy. Who can't exercise for 2 minutes? (If that's you, I apologize). And you'll feel successful, and good about yourself. Take that successful feeling and build on it, with another baby step. Add 2-3 minutes to your exercise routine, for example. With each step (and each step should last about a week),

you will feel even more successful. Make each step really, really small, and you won't fail. After a couple of months, your tiny steps will add up to a lot of progress and a lot of success.

13. **Read About It Daily** – When I lose motivation, I just read a book or blog about my goal. It inspires me and reinvigorates me. For some reason, reading helps motivate and focus you on whatever you're reading about. So read about your goal every day, if you can, especially when you're not feeling motivated. Don't forget to check the 7 Day Bomb Facebook fan page for other people's stories and before and after photos.

14. **Call For Help When Your Motivation Ebbs** – Having trouble? Ask for help. Email us! Join in a conversation on our Facebook fan page; call your mother or best friend! Tell them how you feel and ask them for their advice.

15. **Think About the Benefits, Not the Difficulties** – One common problem is that we think about how hard something is. Exercise sounds so hard! Just thinking about it makes you tired. But instead of thinking about how hard something is, think about what you will get out of it. For example, instead of thinking about how tiring exercise can be, focus on how good you'll feel when you're done, and you'll be healthier and slimmer over the long run. The benefits of something will help energize you.

16. **Squash Negative Thoughts; Replace Them with Positive Ones** – Along those lines, it's important to start monitoring your thoughts. Recognize negative self-talk, which is really what's causing your slump. Just spend a few days becoming aware of every negative thought. Once you catch a negative thought – say "STOP!" Then focus back on point

15 – the end result, thin, happy etc.

My next bit of wisdom for you is:

SLOW DOWN!

Are you a rush-aholic? Always rushing around, trying to cram too much into the little free time we have? No wonder you're failing and not achieving anything. Slow down – just try this!

Doing a task more slowly will produce better results. We've all heard of someone who has burnt out and had a serious health wake-up call like a heart attack to slow down. Slowly, breathe.

Humans need rests, relaxation, and recreation. We need time to think about things, to clear the mind, and to have fun. But to a person overburdened with claims on their time, fun only seems a distant remembered state of mind.

Slowing down is a way to incubate, conserve, and harvest our energy, not about relief from boredom by just watching more TV or going shopping. You may have to confront boredom at first. Sometimes things have to get worse before they get better.

Don't slow down quickly

If you're a rush-aholic and want to slow down, your first impulse may be to try too hard and expect instant results. Making a change takes time and isn't always easy. Expect a period of some discomfort. Many people who retire from an active life feel themselves at a loss. Hyperactivity is often a defense against boredom, and the fear of slowing down is really a fear of confronting yourself.

Workaholism may be the only socially condoned disease. Numerous books have been written about workaholism in America. In Japan there is an expression for death by overwork: Karoshi.

If we let it, work can take over our lives. Work is of course necessary, but the problem is taking it too far. You decide what excess is for you. Having drive is a self-actualizing positive attribute, but being driven, being compelled to work for long-hours, is soul destroying.

It's odd that we have so much material wealth, but so many of us are dissatisfied and unable to enjoy it. When everything is about work we are far less likely to do a good job.

Slowing down has the reward of honoring the unique you, and being present for yourself and others. And what's more, you just may discover the joy in enjoyment. Maybe there is now a new meaning to the phrase slow coach!

So let's put this into perspective as I have two friends both self-employed yet one is always working and the other is always doing social stuff and enjoying life! The one guy works hard all the hours under the sun and the moon to keep his business going, whereas my other friend has a business that works for him, it allows him to enjoy life. If you choose to work long hours (maybe you are self-employed also) then you are in control. But if you work long hours out of fear that if you don't you'll be demoted or fired, then that's a recipe for burnout.

Slowing down, even a small amount, can help you be less demanding, less impulsive, and more patient with yourself and others. If slowing down makes you more considerate of other people, you'll be even more likeable than you are now.

A Thought Experiment

It's your time. It's your life. You can think of time as an investment. So take just a few minutes to imagine now.

Try this thought experiment. If you took tomorrow off and spent it by yourself, what would your day be like? How would you feel? For this experiment you'll do nothing for practical value. You won't use it to get things done.

The above is only a thought experiment. Just thinking about your day, what will the early morning be like? Where will you be at mid-day? Can you describe the place you imagine yourself to be? How do you anticipate your feeling at being alone?

Now try thinking about how you would spend half a day. Remember, this is not time to achieve a goal. You can spend half-day with other people anything you like. How would you feel during this time, and how would you feel afterward?

Slow Hour

If the thought experiment above took only a few minutes, could you actually take an hour to slow down? What would it be like to spend an hour completely free from any pressing matter? We structure our days with every hour taken up – but what about once in a while giving ourselves an unstructured hour between doing things?

The idea behind a lunch hour was that it gave one time for rest, sustenance, and renewal. But this practice has disappeared from many workplaces. Your slow hour could be as easy as assigning importance to this precious time.

Make sure you keep a date with yourself. How would you use your slow hour? Would you be tempted to fill it up with striking things off your to-do list, or would you be able to slow down? Do you have to try it and find out? Would you feel guilty about taking care of yourself?

Slow Calm

More haste, less speed, or haste makes waste are a well-known sayings. When under pressure, the ability to act slowly and deliberately is a benefit. The wise carpenter measures twice and cuts once. Taking time to read the map instead of blindly heading off in what you guess might be the right direction makes sense.

Thinking and considering before acting takes a level of impulse control that's missing when we become overly stressed. Slow is not about being lazy.

Slow Eating

My mum would say don't rush your food! Children eat like animals until they are civilized. We eat and run! The slow food movement started in Italy as a backlash against fast food, but this is another subject. Current wisdom has it that eating slowly can help you lose weight. Taking your time to chew your food releases the nutrients. It's easy to overeat, but slowing down can help.

We often see food as fuel. You are more likely to eat quickly if you live alone. You are more likely to eat quickly if you are working at the same time. When we gulp down our food our stomachs don't have a chance to digest it properly, nor signal to our brains that we are satisfied.

Taking a break between courses or eating smaller portions and waiting, eating with others, and taking time to digest what you eat is a good way to practice slowing down. Turn the TV off and just be mindful of the food before and as you eat it.

Exercise Slow

If you've ever tried to lift weights at the gym, you'll know that doing it very slowly is far more demanding than doing it quickly. The idea of weight lifting is to build muscle. However, it's common to see people rush through their routines counting repetitions, as if more is better. If they went more slowly, and used less weight they would get the result they are after more quickly. Look at yoga, that is all about control, sense, breathing and awareness – you can't rush yoga!

Multi-Tasking

I don't get peoples obsession with boasting about being a great multi-tasker! I am not! It's hard at times not to multi-task but I prefer not to. Our bodies are alive with electro-chemical reactions. We are constantly breathing, thinking, and monitoring our internal and external environments. Yet we can choose to do fewer things in order to concentrate better.

When driving we can choose to drive safely, not to answer the phone, or listen to the radio, or talk to passengers. We can choose to just drive. Slowing down can teach us to notice more of what is going on around us.

Slow Attention

Slowing down helps give our full-attention to what we are doing. Try walking slowly. Pause before responding to questions.

Slow Down Now

Personal energy, attention and time are limited. By slowing down we can use these better to our advantage.

My next bit of wisdom for you is:

6 SECONDS TO RELAX

Smile, breathe and go slowly.

Ever had one of those days when it seems there's not a minute to catch your breath, let alone meditate or relax? A day when you feel like the proverbial busy bee, with no time to admire the fragrant flowers you're landing on?

So what do you do when you have one of these days? Where is there space to stop, slow down and relax? Well on these days could you spare at least 6 seconds?

Yes that's right… **6 seconds**. That's the time it takes to let yourself have 1 relaxing breath. 2 seconds breathing in through your nose, 4 seconds exhaling through your mouth. Right now, I'm going to ask you to take 12 seconds for an experiment. At the end of this sentence, practice that relaxing breath… 2 seconds in and 4 seconds out.

That's right. And once again at the end of this sentence.

Even that little amount of time – 6 seconds – can help your body and mind relax. Let your heart rate slow. Let some of the stress slide away.

Now how can you give yourself the gift of relaxing breaths during even your busiest days? One answer is to pair a relaxing breath with an activity that comes up repeatedly during your day. For example, let's say you're a secretary.

Each time your phone rings, breathe before you answer it.

There should never be a day even your busiest where you cannot take time to just breathe.

My next bit of wisdom for you is:

LOVE LIFE, NOT STUFF

We're in love with stuff – with shopping, with acquiring, with owning, with collecting.

Let's lust after life instead.

Our obsession with stuff has become unhealthy. When we have a void in our lives, we buy things. When we have problems, we buy things. And these things are becoming more and more expensive, bigger, shinier... and more wasteful.

This obsession with stuff leads to owning a lot, having a lot of clutter... and yet this stuff doesn't fill our lives with meaning.

It leads to deep debt, from buying so much, and needing bigger houses and storage spaces to contain everything. Financially, we're worse off than ever, because of this obsession with stuff.

We buy things when we're depressed, we buy things for others to show how much we love them... and in this way, stuff has separated us from actually dealing with our emotions, blocked us from truly connecting with others.

Let's replace that lust for stuff with a lust for life.

Here are some ideas:

- Rediscover a passion for life. Get outside and feel nature, appreciate the beauty of the world around you. Get active, do some gardening, play a sport, go for a walk, take a hike, go for a swim, ride a bike. Feel the life coursing through you. Breathe it in.

- Give experiences as gifts, not stuff. Instead of shopping for someone for a birthday or Christmas, think of an experience you can give them instead. A date with you, doing something fun, hanging out, cooking, playing, talking, exploring. A fun time at a park or beach. Something other than every day. An experience is much more meaningful than an object.

- Connect with others. In real life. If you haven't hung out with a friend recently, give him a call and go hang out. Get your kid away from the TV or video game player and take them outside to do something. Go on a date with your partner, my wife and I take date night once a month. But be present when you're with them – really take time to listen.

- Deal with your emotions. If you have a need to buy things, to shop when you are having emotional issues, be more aware of this. Then deal with the underlying emotions, rather than using shopping as a way to forget about them. If you're depressed, or anxious, or lonely, deal with those. Find solutions; figure out what's causing them. Good news: experiencing life, getting active, and connecting with others all help you deal with those emotional issues.

- Disconnect your attachment to stuff. Sometimes I find myself reluctant to give something up, even if I don't really use it. And that's when I ask myself, "why?" What is holding me back from getting rid of this possession? Sometimes, the item has an emotional connection, but then I realize that it's just an object, it's not the emotion or the actual source of the emotion. Then I'll take a picture of the item, upload it to my computer, and get rid of the object. I feel liberated, because I've broken an attachment to a physical object (but saved the memory). If you are attached to an object, figure out why – it's not healthy in the long run.

- Realize that life, not stuff, is what matters. Objects are just objects – if you lose them, if they get stolen or destroyed… it's not a big deal. They're just objects – not your life. Your life is the series of moments that is steaming through your consciousness right now, and how you use those moments and what you fill them with is what truly matters, not what you fill your home with. At the end of this short journey, you'll look back and remember your experiences, the people you loved and who loved you back, the things you did and didn't do. Not the stuff you had.

Don't forget there will be many more pieces of wisdom on the 7 Day Bomb blog so please follow us there.

REALIZE THIS…

"The purpose of life is a life of purpose" **Robert Byrne**

This is going to be a tough chapter to read for some people but I found this advice transformed my thinking, it made me look at myself and my family in a different light. It made me sit up straight and take a deep breath.

Death. The end of your life. It's always approaching. Every day is a day closer to that day when we leave this life.

I can hear some of you already "come on Scott this is so negative" but wait a second. I am not dwelling negatively on death – yes it is a horrible necessary but it's just a part of life. It's normal, we all experience death through losing loved ones and we will experience it ourselves someday. Let's hope that day is a long way in the future (that comment is for all of those who accused me of being negative!)

But hear me out here; I just want to end this book by

putting everything into perspective. You now have:

1. A 7 day plan where you can lose 7 pounds if you keep the law
2. A few more ideas to help you shed even more such as walking and the shiver system
3. I have even shared with you some mindfulness techniques and some wisdom to help you consider a lifestyle change

But that's all I can do. You are responsible for your life. And so I just want to encourage you now to set the date for your first 7 Day Bomb and get the first 7 pound off.

This time next week you will be 7 pounds lighter.

So let me leave you with this thought to think about as you transform your beautiful life:

WHAT IS THE MEANING OF LIFE?

We can try and provide an answer to this through religion or arguments but it still doesn't satisfy why we, you and me are here. What is our purpose in life?

I have pondered this question for too long, my wife Naomi can testify to this! Then about 12 months ago I realized that (like my quote underneath the chapter heading) it's to <u>live a life of purpose.</u> A life of purpose, purpose to your family, friends, neighbors, work colleagues and your fellow human beings whoever they are.

How can we do this when we are so infatuated with food on the one hand and then dieting on the other? We need balance, control and also health. So this leads me on to tell you getting healthier and dropping excess weight is the number one priority in your life right now alongside working to provide for your family.

Realize this...

Death is coming and you don't realize how little time you actually have left.

If I was generous I would say the average western human being has a good chance of reaching 80 years old in their life.

The first twenty-five years one usually spends growing, learning, studying and most likely adding weight! So we can write these years off. The last 20 years of one's life is spent in old age and sickness, so we can also write these years off. So realistically the average western human being only has about 35 years at the most to do anything worthwhile and of purpose.

Let me demonstrate my life:

I am 32 years old, my useful years left works out to be only 28 years:
80 (Average Life Span) – **32** (Age) – **20** (for old age) = **28** years of purpose

So please don't read this wrong way and get negative and depressed. See this as enlightenment into the reality of what we have left. Once we understand how little time we have left on this planet we can realize the urgency of everything and begin working for the happiness of ourselves and others.

If you are 60 or above then I know your wisdom and life experience won't allow you to be offended by my advice on realizing how little we all have left and that you will agree with this advice for a younger generation.

So use this calculation above to work out your purposeful years left and make it happen.

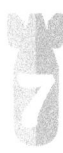

CHANGE YOUR WORLD

Thank you for purchasing the 7 Day Bomb – I really do hope it has given you a refreshed outlook on your life and provided you with the tools to drop 7 pounds at a time. If you do take the 7 day bomb and don't break the law I really do hope you will drop me a mail with your results!

You're a beautiful and truly unique individual who has so much potential inside you. Remember the purposeful time you have left and cherish it with a healthy body and mind.

Happy Everything!

Scott & Nay

7 Day Bomb – Damage Control

MEDICAL DISCLAIMER

7 Day Bomb reflects the authors experiences, knowledge, and expertise; and the information, advice and instruction from same are provided for educational purposes and general reference only; and are not intended to be a substitute for medical, fitness or dietary advice or counseling. Therefore, you should consult your own physician and/or mental health professional regarding your individual physical and mental health needs before undertaking this system, or any other plan, diet, exercise, or fitness program. Results on this plan may vary according to individual efforts and/or other factors beyond the control or expertise of the creator.

The contents of this book, such as text, graphics, images, and other material contained ("content") are for information purposes only. The content is not intended to be a substitute for professional nutrition, fitness or medical advice, diagnosis or treatment. Always seek the advice of your physician or other qualified health provider with any questions you may have regarding a health or medical condition. Never disregard professional advice or delay in seeking professional advice because of something you have seen in this book. None of the content in this book is intended to be instructional for nutrition, fitness or medical advice, diagnosis or treatment.

This book contains articles on many medical/health/nutritional/diet topics; however, no warranty whatsoever is made that any of the articles are accurate. There is absolutely no assurance that any statement contained or cited in an article touching on medical/health/nutritional/diet matters is true, correct, precise, or up-to-date. Even if a statement made about health/nutrition/diet is accurate, it may not apply to you or your symptoms.

The information provided in this book is, at best, of a general nature and cannot substitute for the advice of a professional (for instance, a qualified doctor/physician, nurse, pharmacist/chemist, and so on). 7 Day Bomb is not a doctor, or health professional.

None of the individual contributors, authors, owners, authors of 7 Day Bomb or anyone else connected to 7 Day Bomb can take any responsibility for the results or consequences of any attempt to use or adopt any of the information presented in this book.

END